Quiet in the Tornado:
A Disability Primer

Written by Carrie Dearborn

Savvy Press
Salem, NY

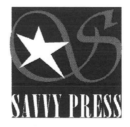

SAVVY PRESS

Published as an imprint of Savvy Press, PO Box 63, Salem, NY, 12865 www.savvypress.com

Book Cover Design: Lisa Dearborn
Interior Design by: Mary Kennedy, LinkPink.com
Bibliography by: Barbara Beckwith
Manuscript preparation: Maida Tilchen
ISBN-13:978-1479103249
ISBN-10: 1479103241

Disclaimer: *Quiet in the Tornado: A Disability Primer* is a resource for persons interested in disability and rehabilitation. Its sole claim is to provide a theoretical perspective, and through a variety of procedures, to introduce interested persons to a process of adaptation. It is not offered as and does not constitute psychological advice. A counselor-client relationship is not established by the use of the content of this book. You should consult a licensed professional regarding any specific issues you have.

Dedication

This is for all those angels out there, especially Mom, Dad, and the woman who has been my caregiver for twenty-seven years.

Table of Contents

Table of Contents continues on next page.

INTRODUCTION

In 1981, when I was fresh out of a coma, my friend read to me. Novels, even short stories, were too long and complicated. It took a long time to find a book that I could understand. What finally worked was a book of collected newspaper columns, by Ellen Goodman of the Boston Globe.

I was barely out of a coma when I tried writing a book. I wanted to create one for newly disabled people. It would have short but interesting articles. Large print. Heavy paper. It could lie flat, but it could be held easily. Or better yet, be on tape. (That was about the extent of technology for disabled people at the time. I discovered early that the technology was there, but ridiculously expensive.)

So here it is, thirty years after I first dreamt it. Someone asked who my audiences would be. Answer: Young people who are newly disabled; Iraq and Afghanistan War vets; people affected by urban industrialism, and the violence that is striking everywhere, not just inner cities; and re-disabled Baby Boomers. These may seem to be so disparate that they have nothing in common, but they really do. Disability used to be a greater leveler than it is now. First it totally devastated your assets, then a completely inaccessible society made it impossible legally, and architecturally to replenish them.

However, I'm not here to depress you with statistics. You have a whole different set of circumstances than I did, and you're often hitting the ground running, so to speak, because there are less attitudinal and architectural barriers to face. Hurray for you!

The first section of this book is specifically for someone who has just gone through an ordeal, as well as his or her friends and family, all of whose lives are now totally upside down. It will be easy to read, and hopefully a little optimistic, but not overly so. I took the liberty of yelling at the annoying things people do to people in comas. I've been waiting thirty years to do that. I hope you don't mind. I'd have appreciated it back then.

For the informative articles in the second section, I hope I produce a team approach. People feel that they have to blame someone. Grudges and guilt arise. Forget all of it. Heal, that's all that matters.

I'm not saying everyone is going to start walking soon, just that no one can predict anything.

The third section gives some ideas on life after disability and the rehab hospital. I think that you, the newly disabled up and coming, will be able to write this better than I can. Just as I stood on the shoulders of the first Disability Rights activists, you'll be able to spring off the hundreds of us dinosaurs and run. I can't wait to see how you do.

Throughout this book, please remember that I've interacted with hundreds of disabled people, although mainly those disabled before the Americans with Disabilities Act (ADA). Unfortunately, many of the "newer" studies of disability presented at conferences use statistics dating back to 1992, when disability was quite different than it is now. There is now a whole generation of people with acquired disabilities who are sort of in the same limbo in which I found myself in 1981: literature less, ideologically bereft, and virtually role-modeless.

In many places, it is much harder now to be as constrained as we were in the 80s, but I don't doubt for a minute that there are still places with no curb cuts, no door openers or accessible busses. I hope this will be useful to younger People with Disabilities [PWD]. Just tolerate me like you do your great aunt. And don't forget your elders! Not only are they the reason you can get on the bus, or roll down the street, but if they get re-disabled, they may experience what you do. So smile!

Don't be lulled by the fact that I use short, non-Latin based words. I took four years of Latin, and if I'm not having a brain blip, I can roughly translate most romance languages. However, my first writing job was for a feminist guidebook, and the fashion of the day was to write to be easily understood. I still agree with that philosophy, although I've revised my opinion that all Latin is unintelligible. It did give rise to some of the largest language groups in the USA: Haitian Kreyol and Spanish.

By the way, one might assume after reading this, that I don't like Harvard Medical or Tufts New England Medical Center. Bite your tongue! Medically, these people are geniuses. They first met me comatose, speechless and paralyzed, and now I'm a loud-mouthed hemiplegic. (My left side is paralyzed.) Their bedside manner needed work, that's all. They are trying, with prodding (and sometimes a legislative slap or two.)

This book allows me to fulfill the one "girl" dream I ever had. When I was young, my father, who was a medic in World War II in Italy (10th Mountain, 86 Division), talked about the brave Red Cross girls who passed out coffee and donuts after the battles. I can't climb mountains anymore, but maybe my words can get to soldiers overseas and here at home. I will be so proud.

Carrie Dearborn
Boston, Massachusetts 2013
Email me at disabilityprimer@aol.com

PART ONE

FRESH OUT OF A COMA

The Physical Therapy walls in my Rehab were dented and marred with gashes. I doubt I drove my wheelchair any worse than anyone else, but from the jokes from the staff, I assumed I was the worst driver ever.

Things might be different now that they've designed usable wheelchairs that can actually move in a straight line. (I'm perfectly serious. My Quickie was the first model to do this, and that was almost twenty years after my stroke!) There are a few things nobody tells the person coming out of a coma; such as:

Who ARE these people? For that matter, who am I? And if I used to smoke, do drugs, or abuse alcohol, for Pete's sake, don't start me again. I'm detoxed if I've been out a week.

What is that thing hanging over my head? A balloon? A mobile? Please take it away. In my coma dreams, to which I'll return shortly, it looks like something that will fall on my head.

Stop yelling for God's sake, and stop asking me so many questions. Last time you asked, I told you the socks go on before the shoes. And there is no earthly reason to flip on the overheads at three a.m. and start talking like it's three p.m.

Did World War 3 start? Brief me please, and don't be surprised if the past year is spotty.

DON'T OPEN THE CURTAINS! MY EYES ARE KILLING ME!

That's enough for now.

FOR FRIENDS AND FAMILY

What not to say, and don't cry. Your loved one needs energy to heal, not comfort you:

1. I know how you feel. (I thoroughly doubt that.)

2. Find joy in what you have. (Yeah, right. I want to grieve now, OK?)

3. Did you ever wish you had just died? (Who ARE you? Satan?)

4. How can you stand this? You used to be so active! (Thanks for the reminder.)

5. I can imagine how you must feel. (I can't hear you yet.).

6. God never shuts a door without opening a window. (So where are these windows?)

7. There's a reason for everything. (Not now.)

8. God never gives you more than you can bear. (There are people this comforts. There are others who can't deal with it right now.)

9. Amazing how people choose their fate. (Excuse me, but are you serious?)

What to say:

10. Too bad you have to go through all this. I brought you a book written just for you. Can I read some to you now?

POSSIBILITIES: AIM HIGH, START LOW

When people at my rehab--visitors, nurses, doctors--found out what I was doing, every single one of them thought I was writing for THEM! Granted, I didn't know that there wasn't anything at the time for them to read, and I felt sort of sorry for them, but the fact remained that they (I thought) could walk away, go home, not be in horrible pain, go to a caregiver group, get sympathy from people...

Ahhh, the grass is always greener on the other side. No one ever told me that they couldn't sleep, they felt lost and isolated, that they were in pain ALL the time. I'm not sure who won out in the end. It has probably evened out by now, but for a long, long time, I think I was less scarred than my friends and family.

Added to all this was the fact that I'd come out as a lesbian two years before the stroke. There was a small group of disabled lesbians writing on disability issues in California, but since nobody on the East Coast knew about it, I felt very alone in that way too. Back then, lesbians were hated even more virulently than disabled people. So much so that the first time I heard someone say disability discrimination, I laughed.

Friends of color have told me that white people always get things wrong. Well, hey, I can see how that can happen. There is a glossing over of certain subjects, like race and disability, so I won't get a clear analysis. I'm not going to pretend racism doesn't exist though. The folks at the Minorities with Disabilities Advocacy Council have been good at clueing me in over the years, and I'll try to pass that information along. The Disability Rights movement has been perceived as mostly white, probably because some people think polio was a white middle-class disease, and that's where the Disability Rights Movement was assumed for a long time to have started. Well, that's not so. Polio hit every race and class, and I'm not convinced that several segments of the population have been heard all throughout history. But enough of the soapbox!

Anyway, from what I'm observing in Boston, there is a huge shift going on. A whole lot of people of color are changing that perception. Not only is environmental racism rearing its ugly head, but more people are getting Medicare and Medicaid assistance. Since home and farm workers have been paying into Social Security (it was the fault of racist legislators that they had been excluded), people of color can get "benefits" and be out and about.

I'm trying hard not to digress, a fault of mine I can't totally blame on my brain damage: I was like that before.

So back to you people with disabilities: Does it seem to you that everyone else is adjusting easily?

Well, forget that idea! Denial is running very high. Your smiling parents and your significant other are crying for hours out of your earshot. Your siblings can't talk about it yet, but have trouble sleeping. Your friends can't visit because they are devastated. Your hospital roommate dreams about suicide, if s/he can dream yet. But everyone is putting on a good face so you can heal.

The first thing to do is GRIEVE!

You have suffered an enormous loss, and you need to grieve. You may need assistance to do this. If you are totally paralyzed, the tears will make your ears itchy, and if you cry very hard, you may choke or get painful spasms. Start out slow.

Of course, when I first came out of a coma, I had aphasia, and so laughed when I wanted to cry, and had no control when it came too slow or too fast. So do the best you can. That's all anyone, including yourself, can expect from you. You may not like yourself very much right now, but trust me, a lot of people do and will like you. Even you, hopefully.

Bear in mind, though, that mostly everyone hates rehab, it hurts a LOT, and you've undergone a huge change. Your body will seem alien to you.

It won't always be like this.

POST-COMA NIGHTMARES AND FRESH LOSSES

Being technically out of a coma, in the realm of the "minimally responsive," was a horrible ordeal. I thought I was having nightmares. I did not understand what was really happening. This is not always the case: my friend Mike went through his coma rather peacefully.

The dream I remember best was the female version of the myth of Sisyphus, and since I never dwelled on Greek mythology, I really don't know why. Some poor young woman plods up a mountain of salt. Just before she gets to the top, the mountain dissolves, and she has to start over.

(Hmm. This wasn't the way I looked at life at all; no wonder I was depressed for so long!)

Anyway, what I was going to say is that fresh loss and exacerbations can be as devastating as the original loss. I found this out many years later when I was told my bladder had to be removed. I was very surprised at my reaction. I got really angry with my doctor of 12 years and said some unkind things. I realized (with uncharacteristic rapidity) that I was repeating a lot of the undesirable behaviors that my disability had originally produced, and resolved to do better. But I had no more control over my emotions than the first time. I burst into tears over the slightest thing. My muscles clenched and released unexpectedly, and I kept thinking people were purposely tricking me.

It's no wonder books and movies skim right over rehab as if it never happened. It's extremely hard to make any sense of it, and painful to write about. Since I've been rewriting these beginning chapters, I've re-experienced the killer claustrophobia, the total uncertainty of anything meaning anything again.

One of the problems of rehab is that there is no respite from it. Friends can take you away for the day if you're lucky, but you must always return. I've since realized that I was blaming an institution for societal mores, which in the '80s, seemed to be: Disabled=ignore her. Stick her in a high crime neighborhood in Boston, along with elderly black people, and whatever you do, DON'T TALK TO HER!

This sort of mindset is less prevalent now, but it has not disappeared. Watch the video of the paraplegic being dumped from his wheelchair, or read stupid Internet jokes mocking people who are different. And disabled literature doesn't always help. If you're feeling down already, reading more of the same isn't exactly fun. Reading *Pollyanna* isn't the ticket either. I don't know about religious books. I had the Berlin Wall erected around my heart. The chaplain, whom I liked, but refused to talk religion with, jokingly (I think) called me "The Heathen."

Being a writer advocating disability rights is a tight-wire act. I don't want to ignore the hard parts, but I don't always feel like that woman plodding up that hill of salt either. I'm aiming for the Barry Corbet style of journalism. Barry produced some hard-hitting pieces, tucked into a glossy magazine, *New Mobility*, which evidently satisfied advertisers.

Being disabled used to mean you could make up your own life because there were no rules to follow and few predecessors to look to. There are more now, but very few people know enough about the subject to tell you who they are. And of course, new people with disabilities are added every day.

One disabled activist who made up not just her own life, but wrote legislation which eases our lives, Connie Panzarino, often said that living well was the best revenge.

Right she was. She delighted in the fact that she outlived several doctors who had her dead and buried. I delight in the fact that the best times in my life were spent in one of the "worst" neighborhoods in Boston, living among other societal outcasts. People who become disabled after the ADA can still find improbable delights. An aphasic man I went to rehab with in the 90s, Rabbi L. Zion, became a poet and relearned Hebrew. I don't know if the Boston street artist, Sidewalk Sam, had all sorts of dire predictions given him, but I'm immensely impressed with his carrying on of his mission.

I used to feel badly for some people at my original rehab. Their families would say, "Why can't you be more like Carrie and talk?" like it was magic or something. I can talk mainly because two friends, Debbie and Joanne, helped me. They had put in a Kirsner button (a special button, which is apparently not still available, but can easily be made by punching air holes in the lavender-size test tube cover and then put on a tracheotomy hole) and spent hours with me while I practiced vocalizing. They researched the latest treatments and wrangled with doctors and nurses.

Well, I've come to the point where my brain damage is pleading with me to stop. It's time for some feel-good stuff.

A RAINBOW FOR THE BLUES: WHY I LIKE WHEELCHAIRS

Do disabled Amazons ever get the blues? If so, what do they do to make themselves feel better?

This has been a long, humid and very hot week. I can't go out because the smog makes me sick and the humidity sets off spasms and pain. It's slowly dawning on me I've had this stupid pain for seven months and if it keeps up, it will mean major changes in my life; plus the fact that even with the air conditioner on high, it is still hot.

I needed escape, so I worked on this article. My tentative title is "Why I Like Wheelchairs," although I hope I can get more imaginative than that.

So, here are my thoughts on "Why I Like Wheelchairs:"

1. They're a good crowd barometer.
I never noticed this until I got lost in a crowd who'd come
to see Winnie and Nelson Mandela. Back in the '80s,
people in a crowd usually stepped all over me, walked in
front of me, and/or made rude comments. None of that in
this crowd. They stepped aside; people of all races. I'd
never have understood how remarkable the Mandelas
were until I'd experienced that minor miracle.

2. I can go leisurely past construction sites now.
No embarrassing remarks. Those big, burly guys treat me
like their aunt or their mother. I like that now, even
though I resented it very much for years.

3. People tend to notice you even if you don't notice them.
This comes in handy, especially if you live in a big city.
Say you're sitting waiting for a bus and get caught in the
rain with no umbrella. Someone who noticed you at a
meeting might come along and put an umbrella over you.
This sort of help is great in a large city, where it once took
me half an hour to get help ringing a doorbell.

4. Other people in wheelchairs almost always say hello to
other people in wheelchairs, depending on how
"individualist" people think they are in that state. It's like
being in a club, or what the early '80s were like when

more gay people 'looked' gay and often winked at each other.

When someone is newly disabled, most people send sympathy cards. I sent one person a congratulation letter instead, telling him to be glad to be part of such a caring group of people.

5. The electric ones are fast (like my Quickie.)
Nothing to be sneezed at when you're sick and have very little energy to begin with. Also, you can go shopping with averagely-abled friends. They get tired before you do. Or, for instance, when a friend of mine was in a hospital, I visited him a lot. Thanks to having a wheelchair that goes 7 mph, it took me no time at all to get there, and I wasn't the least bit tired.

6. The newer ones actually make you feel sexy.
Feeling sexy may be a tough one to swallow, but if you'd suffered through eight years of being uncomfortable and in pain, you'd feel human in a chair that makes no noise, is comfortable, and can go across a busy city street safely, with enough speed to get you to the other side before the light changes. (Especially my Quickie, which had the first skirt guard I'd ever had on a chair! Until then every dress I wore got ruined. I've never been much of a clotheshorse, but occasionally, I like to dress.)

7. Finally, I also like wheelchairs because they're great babysitters. I once sat next to a fussy two-year-old at a meeting. I unplugged my horn, taped the on/off switch and let him play. Not a peep out of him for two hours, which is unbelievable for so young a child. I took him for a slow ride after the meeting, too. Then I had to leave, which, seeing as he tried pushing my chair back into the room, he seemed quite reluctant to let me do.

Babies and toddlers think wheelchairs are delicious and wonderful jungle gyms. Words of warning, though. First, wash your wheels and rims with ammonia, and then rinse with water. Secondly, don't let them teeth your chair unless you like little tooth prints on your rims. Lastly, drive SLOWLY and VERY CAREFULLY. Always double check that there's no child behind you before you back up.

Have fun with children. Even if you're a whispering quad, have someone place a baby on your lap and just think love. The toddler will turn to you, grin, and then pull your hair. I know. I tried.

GOD'S WINDOWS EXPLAINED: DEALING WITH FEELINGS OF GLOOM AND DOOM

One day Connie Panzarino (lifelong activist for people with disabilities) and I were sitting around, talking about things people say about disability. We went through a few truly silly ones (see "For Friends and Family") and got around to "God never shuts a door without opening a window." She said it was more like God put a great big accessible garage door there, complete with a door opener. Not an itsy bitsy window.

That may be hard to swallow right now. I know that when I was in rehab, getting through the next minute was about all I could handle. Breathing was hard enough. I know not everyone is in that amount of pain, and not everyone has the amount of brain damage I did. But I do know that your Physical Therapy is exhausting you. They don't call it Pain and Torture for nothing!

You don't need to figure out where the darn windows are right now anyway. Looking back at my rehab days, the only thing I can see, as far as hidden windows that only disabled people can find, is that violent 'lunatics' (the psych ward was around the corner) would not hurt me. They tried to hurt the staff, yes, but not me.

And I kept trying to figure out the "reason" I was in a wheelchair, a totally pointless waste of time that lasted ten years until I finally realized it didn't matter. All the reasons people came up with back then with did not at all fit. It was really annoying to be told I went through all that pain just "so they could be inspired by me."

Oh yes, there's one more hidden window. As a professional athlete, I never had to suffer that demoralizing gradual loss of ability. I probably peaked at 20, when I became a certified ski instructor, but during my last year of skiing (at age 27) I noticed my short swing was not as precise as it had been. I didn't have to live through that gradual decline. Nope, my body was almost in top form when it failed completely. And it's given me a lot of pleasure over the years to just keep that one to myself.

So your body wasn't so great before? You can still find a way of looking at things that will give you secret pleasure. I used to wonder how people with progressive diseases could deal with things, so I asked some people. Turns out I was seeing things with a doom and gloom outlook. Instead of seeing just pain and death because of my chronic kidney disease (which fortunately, I didn't know about at first), I needed to understand that it would force me into knowing some quite remarkable people. Also, that

I would cherish those seconds of painlessness I usually experienced. (But sure didn't when I tried to pass a kidney stone!)

Some people are glad they had certain abilities for as long as they did. Others are glad they learned coping mechanisms years before the aging population does. (Really, it's quite funny to hear aging friends start complaining about forgetfulness, when you've been coping with it for years.) I guess if you're lucky enough to become old, being slightly disabled isn't too far from the regular course of things. Of course, many older people don't agree.

See? Things will work out, they are definitely NOT as bad as it seems. Forget Jerry Lewis and telethons saying we're half a person. There will be times you'll feel like your old self.

OK, FEEL GOOD TIME: HEROES AND SHEROES TO INSPIRE US

One of the smartest men in the world, Stephen Hawking, uses a wheelchair. At least three Cambridge, Massachusetts, universities (MIT, Harvard, and Cambridge College) are equipped with door openers, presumably in case he ever wants to drop by. (This sounds like a joke, but you'd be surprised at the effects you will have on people who see you struggle with obstacles or other inaccessible things. I was the inspiration for two automatic door openers myself, and I'm no Stephen Hawking.)

Well, hey! We've been around a while, we disabled women and men, and not just white people either. My personal favorite is Harriet Tubman, who suffered seizures from her early teens. It didn't stop her from saving a lot of slaves via The Underground Railroad, now did it? Exactly how many is debatable, but at least 100. She did, apparently, sleep right through a slave revolt she was supposed to help. That tidbit of news allowed me to feel OK about the frailty of my body when I miss something really important.

People in comas, physically disabled people, and people with mental illnesses are not always scorned or spit upon. Sometimes it seems like we are and always have been. I seem to remember a period, actually, quite a long period, in which I kept seeing scenes from German Holocaust movies in which we got shot or were forced to beg. But then I did a workshop with newly arrived Bostonians. It was the culmination of a yearlong health care project with many immigrants, and from the nonjudgmental eager questioning, I realized not all cultures were heartless as that one was. (And if my father, a World War II medic, could like current day Germans, then so can I.)

Uh Oh. This is a brain damage tip. Sometimes your writing or speaking seems to devolve to the point where nothing seems related to anything else. Just shut your mouth or stop writing at that point, and don't worry about making sense. Friends tell me it will, especially to other brain damaged people. (I read a *Science News* article in which medical students described our speech as "gibberish." Guess they never listened to themselves!)

And if you feel really unredeemable and stupid, like I have, well forget it!

Here's a little piece I wrote years ago. It's sappy, and I wrote it for the money, which I never did get, but it crystallizes a longer article later in this book.

CALLING ALL VEGETABLES: SURPASSING LOW EXPECTATIONS

Fourteen years after my stroke, I was in a state senator's office explaining why the ten per cent cap on housing for people with disabilities seemed discriminatory. The senator was engrossed in what I was saying, and all I could think was "Hey! Not bad for a vegetable!"

I became an advocate for a disability group, intending only to fill in for a few weeks, but somehow I ended up staying for three legislative seasons. It was volunteer work, but a rehab would have charged thousands to teach me that I could do this much.

In 1981, I was told that I'd never be more than a vegetable, and somewhere deep down, I believed this. Don't ask me why. They'd been wrong about nearly everything else: I came out of the coma, I talked, I regained use of my limbs, and I'd even regained my ability to write fiction. Somehow, though, I figured I'd never surpass what I'd already done.

Before my stroke in 1981, I'd been a computer operations specialist at a time that the industry was 95 percent white male. Months before my stroke, my manager left and I became responsible for overseeing the flow of cash from 43 theatres. It took me years and years to accept the fact that those management skills were now beyond my reach. Turns out they were there, but the ability to transmit the signals wasn't.

The disability advocacy job forced me into doing things all my neuropsychology tests said were impossible: decision making, prioritizing, problem solving. These were agonizingly slow at first, especially since they had once been so easy for me. What probably kept me trying, and believe me, there were many times I wanted to give up, was that no one at the agency would let me. Every person there had exceeded all expectations people had for them too. I probably could have shared my problems more, but that's a bit much to ask of an over-institutionalized person.

The thing I did not understand and I may have been told, but did not get, was that my brain was so impacted by the stroke that I had to retrain my brain in the complexities too. Not just the simple stuff, like reading, writing and arithmetic, but the harder things too. Writing books or designing work flow systems may come eventually, but definitely not right away. It does get easier, once you get over the hump thinking it is impossible. It's actually quite exciting. You never know what you will come to remember the next day. (I regained sensory memories, the absence of which made me feel like an impostor.)

Working with people who expect you to function well, if unorthodoxly, is a huge boost to your self-esteem. Years and years of not being able to do the simplest things, of thinking I was unemployable, (and thus would always be in poverty) had sunk me into an unimaginable depression.

Afterthought

At the time I wrote this, I had no clue as to how incredibly hard it is to find an employer willing to hire a disabled and older worker. There are smart and legislatively effective people working on this problem, and if I keep up my end of this collective bargaining unit we call society, I can count on them to hold up theirs.

LIFE THREATENING DISEASE ISSUES

During the 80s and half of the 90s, hundreds of my friends and acquaintances died of AIDS. I once tried to count and gave up somewhere in 1986 when I hit 50. Mine was not a unique situation either. Everyone I knew was either going to a hospital or a memorial service.

Writing articles sort of fell by the wayside. Supporting People with Disabilities--including AIDS--was what people I knew were doing. I had time to write a few articles, but I didn't always submit them. Because they were written when my brain damage was relatively fresh, I made these amazing leaps, sometimes mid-sentence. I doubt I can edit them to make more sense to non brain damaged people.

In any case, they address some of the issues not just for dying people, but for people living with life-threatening illnesses. The circumstances of AIDS have completely changed! With the new meds, it is simply a chronic disease. There are some things only an AIDS or HIV educator can tell you about, but any disability has specialists.

A BURDEN?: GETTING OUT OF THE GUILT AND BURDEN TRAP

At his hospital bedside, one of his friends asked me if he had had a chance to talk about death. Well, of course he had, but at the time, I could only remember one conversation he'd had with me, during which I think he finally understood that I didn't think, and probably no one else either, thought of him as a BURDEN.

That one took me years to learn. I used to feel guilty ALL the time. I had ruined my former lover's life--she'd quit school when I had the stroke. One brother slid further into depression. My parents stopped going to church. I was a BURDEN. I should just die and be done with it. People think you can do that. I have no doubt some people can, but it's hard to do. Believe me, I know.

But that's what he wanted to do: lie down and die.

Besides, that being fairly impossible to do, he needed to examine this idea that he was a burden.

To whom, exactly? Not one of his legions of friends had ever said that. Almost all of them had told me they wanted to know more about him. Me? As his 'sister', I had as much obligation as anyone, but I CHOSE to stick by him.

That people had freely chosen to care for me were magic words back then. I hadn't made anyone do anything. They had chosen their reactions.

Before he died, Mike told me he felt mostly guilty about me. I tried to find out why - he was uncharacteristically unclear. I finally settled on telling him that I chose to stick around.

I think it worked. During his last year, I thought I was constantly messing up, but during his last week at the hospital he couldn't have been more loving. Even when he was mostly unresponsive, he flashed beatific smiles at his friends' greetings.

I don't think a person who thinks he's a burden does that.

HOW TO ALMOST DIE: and WHY YOU SHOULD STAY ALIVE

(Originally written during the worst years of AIDS.)
First of all, relax! The first minute is wonderful, that's all I can tell you from experience, but my gut feeling is that it stays that way. The first thing that indicated that I was dying (although since I never was taught this, I messed up a great death) was that I floated to the ceiling. From up there, I watched with great interest just what was happening to my body and my friends. Although right before I passed out, I told my lover "right side of brain, left side of body", I thought that I was having a heart attack. I saw my lover and our friend looking worriedly at my body and I wished they knew I was okay.

At this point, I should have seen that light in front of me and headed straight for it. But I was too busy looking back, feeling awful leaving my lover. No great voice told me to go back. (Author's note: I have since learned that some stroke patients do not get to see the light. Rats, huh?)

This is when the ambulance people came. I assume they did things to revive me. But for years, I blamed my lover for keeping me here. It may have been that, but I know part of it was that I'd never been taught how to die right. And my lover had not been taught how to let go. As a result, two people who once had a dream relationship were now scared to even touch.

Death is not a subject some North Americans speak about very much. Neither is disability. Consequently, some of us do both of them badly. Well, I want to discuss death here, because I suffered so badly after I bungled my own.

When you come out of your body, you may be dying, or you may simply be escaping pain. (I used to do this and I was no expert on out-of-body experiences.) If you are dying, you will just be able to feel that something special is happening. This is where the lover or the family can help. You may think you're dumb and untrained in these things, but you know a lot more than you think. You may actually hear your lover's voice in your mind, or you may hear a change in breathing. While you are waiting for help to arrive, wave to your lover. Doing this helps your lover or family member leave, but it may not be enough.

Talk about death before it happens. I wish I had done this with my 'brother' before he died. I'd had some very serious talks with him about life and death, but since I argued for life, I never got to tell him that it's okay to die naturally. He died a few minutes after I left, after my having been there all day. Sometimes I feel bad about that.

I did get to tell my third close friend who died from AIDS that I wanted him around for selfish reasons, but I loved him too much not to let him go whenever he thought he'd had enough. He received that very enthusiastically, told me people usually saved kind words for funerals instead of telling the person directly.

But, of course, you probably won't be dying tomorrow. Just in case you were thinking of it, below are reasons to stick around.

1. Because not everyone can lie down and die, even if that's all they think about day and night.

I've been told several times that my chances of staying alive were slim. There doesn't seem to be a lot of rhyme or reason to my survival that I can see; I'm no more special than any of the hundreds of writers who have died of AIDS, or my fellow disabled peers, and to suggest it is nauseating to me.

Ten years of pondering this 'reason' thing has led me to believe that machines probably kept me alive. God invented those machines, I'll concede now, but it was mostly machines and private health insurance. My recovery was, at the time, miraculous. That I got back my voice, a lot of my memory, use of one hand and foot, these were miracles. But that was only because I was one of the first AVMS (Arterial Venus Malformation) kept alive. A few years later, 50% of AVMS survived and regained all kinds of abilities.

2. Because you might survive a suicide attempt, and if you think you're in hell now, just wait!

What's kept me from suicide is that I lived next to a locked psych ward for nine months. And I know I'd have to live in one (or the modern equivalent) if I lived through a bungled attempt. Have you been to one lately? You'd think that most of the abuses would be outlawed.

However, there are always new ones popping up that are perfectly legal.

3. Because we want you around, but not if you only suffer.

I hope we're not THAT selfish. We don't care if we have to slow down sometimes. I mean, where are we going? Same place your body is. That article, that book, that business deal will probably get done. If it doesn't, so what? AIDS and other immune system diseases have made me realize that friends and family are far more important than work.

4. Because the year you think will be your last will be incredibly sweet. You won't want to miss it. In the middle of a holiday party, you'll realize this may be the last time you'll do this. All of a sudden, your senses sharpen and every interaction becomes more meaningful. But do pay your taxes and buy a few new pieces of clothing at the end of the season sales. Just in case.

PART TWO

This section is for the person with new disabilities who has been out of a coma for a few weeks, and is facing what seems to be a daunting amount of Rehab, or for someone facing an undetermined hospital stay for another disabling condition.

Oh, I remember both experiences quite well, and in both cases was helped by someone named Nancy.

The first Nancy was a kind young nurse in our rehab who remembered her promises, never secured my wheelchair brakes which would have grounded me, and learned finger spelling, unlike all the other nurses. I could extol her virtues all day, but just by her being kind and trying to communicate with me, I learned that there are good parts in every rotten day.

The second Nancy was a middle-aged nurse whom I met after my bladder surgery. I had stopped eating and drinking for two reasons. One, one of the few friends I had during my bed-bound and very ill days, Mike Riegle, (an early prison and gay rights activist) was showing early signs of AIDS. He was my ears, eyes and legs. And two, in 1988, I was still at risk for AIDS myself, having had a blood transfusion in 1981.Things seemed very hopeless then. Everyone, so it seemed, was dying.

And if that weren't enough, everything I ate or drank ripped right through me. I'd been told my care would get easier, but this cut into the bit of independence I'd carved out.

Enter Nancy, who listened to everything, and told me all I needed to think about was healing, that even if my friend had AIDS, and maybe he didn't, I'd need to be strong and healthy so I could help him.

Turns out he did have AIDS, but I did get healthy and strong. I wished I could have done more, but PWAs used to have to start letting go of life, so probably what I could do was enough.

Anyway, here's the how-to section of the book. It is possible to make a Bloody Mary out of the tomatoes life has thrown at you. (You'll get sick of lemonade. I think they make Virgin Bloody Mary's.)

AFTER HOURS WORK: SORRY!

One night, after all my therapies were done, I went with friends to the vending room. I sat at the table, happily awaiting my M&M's, but to my dismay, they wanted ME to tangle with the vending machine!

"I can't do that" I informed them. They answered that they knew that, but they'd show me.

I don't recall my exact reaction then, but even now I remember my anger and outrage. I deserved some time off, after all!

Well, wrong.

What is this anyway, a two year old talking???

Nearly thirty years later, I'm extremely grateful that I can use a vending machine. A lot of disabled people can't use them or are afraid of them.

What I'm sadly informing you is that you will get no rest for a while. It really stinks. I don't know what to tell you. I know that for years people told me my 'purpose' was to educate people!

I hated that. Still do. It may be true, but I want to participate in life as much as I can, have some fun while I'm here. To do that in the future, here's a suggested list of After Hours Work. I hope you'll forgive me.

1. Cell phones: make sure to put a loose blanket on your lap, because I guarantee you'll drop it. They're slippery! Don't worry if the buttons seem too small, and you can't see the thing very well. They do have ones you can read.

My hands stopped shaking constantly AFTER I got off the medication that was supposed to quiet my shaking. (A medical student had put me on it without my knowledge.) I am constantly amazed that my fine motor skills ever work. Don't disregard technology the way I have, because you never know.

2. Cameras: I simply can't do it. The cameras I learned on were held to the eye, and now they aren't. See what I mean about not letting technology get away from you?

3. Wallets: open and close them, try putting bills and change away. You'll feel good when you can do this. On those days (in the future) when every bill or receipt sticks or crumples, just smile sweetly and remember that those impatient 30-something's will someday get old and sick, if they live that long.

4. Clean hearing aids, glasses: your PCA will get paid to do this, which is great because on a daily basis, it will eat up your day to do everything. But in an emergency, or when

your PCA is out, you should be able to clean your glasses and change your hearing aid batteries. It used to be impossible for me to even attempt changing batteries, but the manufacturers are making it easier. Just put a pillow on your lap and don't pull off that orange sticky thing until the battery is in place.

5. Put on Chap Stick or creams and lotions. I don't know a whole lot about makeup, but I suppose you better stay away from mascara and eye shadow. A blind friend who had severe ataxia wouldn't even touch a dressing stick, although another friend even more ataxic since birth, but not blind, did all sorts of things no one would ever believe.

Even if you are a rugged guy who never uses anything, you may start having to pay attention to your skin. Bedsores are no joke, and if you get one the skin gets less and less able to heal. Bedsores get a lot of us in the end, pun intended.

6. Try cleaning out your handbag (or "Man bag.") Decisions are really hard for some of us, and you'll need practice. Have a friend on hand when you do this, because brain damaged people have been known to discard brand new things.

HOW TO HAVE FUN IN THE HOSPITAL

First off, forget wheelchair races. I tried this once. Don't ask me whose brilliant idea it was to let a child who couldn't see over my handles steer me down a hallway littered with carts and gurneys. I landed on the floor. Good thing I had young bones.

The trick is to let off steam safely without terrifying the nurses and doctors. This isn't easy, but it is doable. Unfortunately, a lot of what you want to do is going to be perceived as unsafe. Once you get out of the hospital, you'll be able to test your limits, but you can't right now. Sorry.

1. Sit at the Nurse's Station, but stay away from the desk. An added attraction is that the elevators are nearby, which means that everyone must pass by. Sometimes this feels creepy to me, especially when the known gossips are out, but it is good to get out of your room, even if it takes three people to move all your machines.

2. A strange game we played for the kids was to put a doll's head on the elevator and send it to the lobby. Then the visitors would come up, the door would open, and there was the doll head. This just delighted the younger patients; it became a fun game of peek-a-boo.

3. My favorite, though, was Washcloth Baseball. The nurses rolled up washcloths and taped them shut. Then they took two tongue depressors and taped them together to make bats. More washcloths made bases. We set up our baseball diamond by the Nurses Station. The visitors enjoyed watching, many tossing us the ball when the elevator doors opened at an inopportune moment.

MISCELLANEOUS THINGS

DO NOT pull what I mistakenly assumed was a friendly courtesy alarm to open the bathroom door. Instead, several nurses charged in, all in full crisis mode, probably with jangled nerves from too much adrenaline.

No food fights. If your dining room is anything like ours, you won't need this to entertain yourself. Just watching the other inmates try to eat will amuse you. That is, if you aren't too busy concentrating on finding your own mouth. (I joke around here with full knowledge that I looked idiotic myself.)

Fantasies are fine, aren't they? So what if your room-mate thinks she lives in Malibu?

It's better than a smelly hospital.

Is there a lounge, sunroom, music room? Go there. Watch the fish swim. If you are able, talk with visitors about anything but yourself. Remind yourself that there is a world out there to which you will probably return. Forget dying, a lot of people can't turn their face to the wall and slip away.

For Halloween, dress up as a vegetable.

The more staid doctors may not think this is very funny. Your nurses probably will.

Another thing you can try entails getting your night nurse to paint your face in washable paint. Polka dots are fine. Have fun keeping a straight face during rounds.

There is a Dorothy Parker quote, of which I have seen several versions. Basically, she tells us to "eat, drink and be merry, for tomorrow we may die, but alas, we probably won't."

HOSPITAL FOOD: AVOIDANCE TIPS

Believe it or not, there are some institutions where the food actually tastes good, is cooked in a healthy way, and is well presented. Unfortunately, this is not always the case, so I'm giving you a run down of various tips I've heard and tried.

Keep in mind that I'm assuming that you've started eating, learned to swallow, and can differentiate between salt and sugar now.

1. Eat out of containers. (Originally suggested to me by a prisoner who was finding strange things in his food.) In some hospitals I might also do this, especially with food allergies. I don't equate hospitals with prisons NOW, but they are both institutions, and survival techniques for one sometimes work fine in the other.

2. Forget eggs and toast. They congeal and get soggy or gloppy. Thank my mother, a retired RN, for this piece of advice. Of course, if you luck out and get a hospital that delivers room service style, and there are some, completely ignore me about pancakes.

3. Eat Kosher. (They have to prepare it with fresh foods. But with a last name like Dearborn, this requires a little chutzpah. I was sort of a Shabbat Goy, so I could at least justify it. Drawback: no ham.)

Gifts to give patients (but only if they have been cleared by the doctor)

1. Buy a metal mesh basket like the picnic napkin holders they sell in the summer. If you can afford it, go to the health food store and buy parsley, mint and dill. Organic herbs are softer than other herbs, and these three herbs will help with digestion. (But skip the parsley if the patient forms kidney stones, and skip mint if heartburn is a problem.)

2. Buy a pepper mill that fits in the napkin holder. Fill it with organic pepper seed.

3. Instead of flowers, see if they sell herb kits. The more organic, the better, but sometimes you can't win. Go to your friends' room and set it up. And try to oversee the watering. I got several pretty arrangements, but many died because the florist had grouped plants with vastly different watering needs, and only the drought tolerant survived.

4. Go to a very cheap vegetable store and buy the cheapest clove of garlic you can find. (The cheaper the garlic, the less growth retardant hormone.) Then separate the clove and press some into the soil if there is a plant in the room. It will send up a fast growing shoot, which can be cut and used for flavor.

HOW IT (USUALLY) WORKS: WHO'S WHO IN THE HOSPITAL

After nurses had switched on the overhead lights at 3AM for the zillionth time, my friends taped the light switch. The very next morning, a totally pissed off woman entered my room, tore off the tape, and snarled, "If you have a complaint, tell the nurse manager!"

Thing is, I really thought I had. Turns out I'd been complaining to the wrong people all along. It didn't help that none of them except Nancy could communicate with me. (In Massachusetts, two organizations with which I worked fought for and got American Sign Language interpreters in hospitals. Please do this elsewhere.)

Anyhow, I learned not to waste my breath complaining to people who can't do anything about the situation. And I saved myself a lot of frustration (when you aren't constantly thinking about a troubling situation, you have room to think about something else.)

My impulse is to start with a supervisor or manager, but I'm really impatient. You won't win friends and influence people this way, and you may run into a manager who has hit the limits of her or his expertise. A lot of unpromoted people will surprise you pleasantly.

When making a complaint, try not to sound judgmental or impatient. (Ha. I need to take my own advice.) Of course, if your speech is garbled, people will make their own assumptions. Not much you can do about that.

So here is a simple organizational chart for Primary Care Nursing, the only method I know personally, the parts that pertain to the patient anyhow.

It is generic. Not every hospital follows it.

Nurse Manager: Co-ordinates the nurses and the day-to-day life of the hospital infrastructure.

Hospital Advocate, or Patient Liaisons: Co-ordinates things like discharge planning, problems the patient faces with Medicare, SSI, etc. Works closely with the social worker and your Primary Care Nurse. (Your first complaint person).

Physical Therapist (PT), Occupational Therapist (OT), Speech Therapist, Respiratory Therapist, Social Worker: Your therapists are probably working together as your rehab team. Any one of them can help you with another discipline. If you are very lucky, you may have a movement therapist.

Registered Nurses: Distribute medications, co-ordinate between patient and doctor, Rehab Therapists, the kitchen, and nursing aides.)

Licensed Practical Nurses, Nurses' Aides, PCAs, CVAs, Orderlies: Wash you up, clean you out and otherwise get you and your bed ready for the day. These are the people you will probably see the most. Brighten up their day. Talk about TV, kids, sports.

People are really funny, but don't give themselves credit. People-watching is something everyone has in common. Joke around with them.

Kitchen staff, housekeeping: By putting up a little rainbow or American flag, a stuffed animal, or pictures of you before all this, let people get a small glimpse of what you're like. You won't believe the favors and stories it will gather.

Some hospitals have volunteer interpreters and sunshine ladies and gents who sell newspapers, playing cards, stationary, distribute juice and donated books.

Maybe because I'm a writer, I notice that more people spill their guts when you are disabled than when you aren't. At least they do in face to face meetings. Then they'd clam up again the minute a "normy" showed up. The ADA has changed this. People actually talk to us now, even in the company of a non-disabled person. I have trouble getting used to this.

Anyhow, the spilling of guts to a disabled person, or non-person, as was probably the case, was a huge boon to my writing. It will probably help you understand your coworkers and colleagues.

PATIENT'S BILL OF RIGHTS – MY VERSION

Back in the olden days, like in the 90s, there was no patient's bill of rights like there is now in Massachusetts. I tried working on one, but couldn't keep it from being too personal.

I still can't, but that's OK. Here is a bill of rights I could have used coming out of a coma in a 1950s mindset environment, one that didn't intend to be that way, but was. Some of the things seem quite obvious, but when you have brain damage and you're on drugs, nothing seems quite real.

1. The doctor works for you, not vice versa. You are a team!

At our independent living center, which I'm told is the second in the country, we disabled people stopped even talking to doctors for a very long time. So many of us had suffered so badly in their hands that it was hard not to run them over. This changed, at least in Boston. By the time I left the Independent Living board, in 1998, there was a stab at--gasp!--working with one.

2. You know your body the best. If, for example, the Phenobarbital you're on to prevent another seizure makes breathing very hard, and you've never had a seizure in your life, ask the doctor to prove you need it. Medical students love to put you on medications whether or not you need them. Some are addictive and make you lethargic. (On the other hand, you may be in denial that you had heart failure and you really need those meds you hate.)

3. Listen to one doctor or nurse you trust and understand. Try not to let the others get you down. The wild guesses and stupid speculations of medical students can make you feel like a neurotic moron! But you usually can tell the

difference between gas and a kidney spasm if you're a hemiplegic!

4. Remember, everything feels different now. You will eventually learn in what ways you were affected, but for now, everything is strange.

WHAT TO ANTICIPATE: SMALL JOYS

No one ever told me anything good would ever happen. People see only losses. True, there has been a lot of loss, and no one is guaranteed any return. I remember hearing--remember, this was 29 years ago--that 90 per cent of stroke patients walk again. I figured I was home free. My mother had beaten the odds twice (polio and being hit by a truck), so I would too. Well, I'm still waiting for my balance to improve.

In the meantime, one has to find fun wherever possible, so here are a few things to look forward to:

Ice Cream!
For some unknown reason, I craved this when I first got out. Be warned though, lactose intolerance sometimes happens to people with chronic illnesses later in life. Try some ice cream before you leave the hospital.

Friends and Family!
You may not know who they are, but you'll probably be able to feel friend or foe. Just keep your mouth shut. They'll fill in the silence, usually with hints.

Freedom!
Long hospital stays and the solitary confinement of a private room and the solitary work of coma rehab lead to a curious condition shared by prisoners: the sheer joy of being free.

Interior Design!
Hopefully, you won't be faced with feces on the walls and cockroach infestations as I was in the 80s. I still live in public housing, and those are in the past, at least in my building. These days, they clean and paint with nontoxic chemicals. Interior design used to intimidate me, but someone from a homeless shelter showed me how to do it. It's not hard.

Attention!
True, sometimes the stares get to be a bit much, especially at first. However, it has gotten a hell of a lot easier for those of us in wheelchairs. I recently got reminded of how bad it used to be. I was chatting with a

friend who is just a little person, and a girl ignored me to stare at her. (Usually I'm the first thing stared at.)

You can turn this around and figure they are staring because you are beautiful. Of course, if you were beautiful before, it may be really difficult to do this. Trust me though, to some people, you are.

BRAIN DAMAGE: JOURNAL OF MY FIRST POST-COMA YEARS

The following is a journal I kept during the 1980s about my own struggles with my brain damage. It has gone through a couple of name changes, but I like plain old "Brain Damage." I've come to love it, this peculiar brain of mine. Granted, at times it frustrates me, especially on hot and humid days when I just cannot find a word or a name, but I keep learning new ways of coping.

Brain Damage 4-9-86

The worst information I got about brain damage was around pain. My brain had swelled and was pressing against my skull. The pain was excruciating. I told one of my nurses about it and she said that "some people learn to live with their pain." I wanted to die right then. I was dizzy all the time (I still am because I have inner ear -

damage). The non-aspirin pain reliever didn't come close to touching the pain. The Phenobarbital they had me on made me dizzier. What no one told me was that the pain would lessen. It took years, but one day I woke up and realized I was only dizzy. I sometimes feel that maybe I am in pain, but because it's nowhere near as bad as that head pain was, I don't count it.

4-10-86

Of all my disabilities, and there are quite a few, the brain damage is both the hardest to understand and the hardest to accept. It's also a hidden disability. I find those harder to cope with than those others can see. People open doors for my wheelchair, yet they may not see that I don't understand and re-explain. A regular conversation, just one you might have over coffee, used to be impossible for me. Not only did I have problems hearing, seeing, and speaking, but I couldn't understand things either. For seven months, I had no voice, so I had to develop other ways to communicate.

Since my vision was so poor and I couldn't turn my head to see who was there, I needed other ways to sense people. I don't know how it happened, but I got good at telling who was there. People can be identified many ways. The easiest is by their foot steps or they'll give themselves away by a yawn or a cough. But some people with vision impairments have another way of sensing that is less easy to explain. To say it's like reading minds is too simplistic, but it's the closest I can come. Some people did say that they could hear my voice talking to them. (Interesting! I had no voice.) Sometimes I could hear their voices without them having spoken, although this was less frequent because my friends could just talk with me. There was nothing wrong with their voices. The most common occurrence was less clear than hearing voices. I knew the other person was there, or thinking of me, or even attempting to tell me something, but it was like trying to understand sign language when you don't know it. You know there's meaning there, but you just can't figure it out.

4-22-86

I lost a lot of IQ points, not that I ever believed they mean much, but I did think of them as a sort of guide. This horrified me at first. Then a vocational counselor told me that all brain-damaged people tested out badly at first and then the number goes back to close to the old one. Sure enough, that's what mine did two years after the insult. I'm very glad it did, but there were certain kinds of thinking I just couldn't do, and that puzzled me.

With brain-damaged people there are all sorts of different kind of thinking going on. Some people can play chess, yet not be able to read. Knowing this, you won't be surprised to know I was re-learning how to think without always using short declarative sentences, but I was also frustrated by my inability to write fiction and do math. I couldn't do the type of combination logic/creative thinking needed for designing systems for computers or writing books.

Part of that frustration was that no one explained to me that all grieving people have very short attention spans: part of it was because my eyes rolled around and I kept losing my place.

4-26-86

I don't exactly know why, but I've just been scared lately. I think it has to do with being able to do that more complex creative kind of thinking. It's a matter now of bringing my body up to the standards of my brain, and I don't know if I can. I've let my body go in some ways, for various reasons, but one of them was that I felt like the brain damage was so bad, it would never repair itself.

I felt this most when I got back the ability to write fiction. I could only write a paragraph. "What good is a paragraph?" I thought. I may as well not have gotten the ability to write fiction back. I couldn't write longhand anyway, so I couldn't write notes and scenes away from my typewriter, which is the way I used to write. Ideas would occur to me at night, at work, on the subway, and I'd write them down. My whole way of being a writer was broken beyond repair, I thought, and I just didn't care to keep trying to write longhand, write fiction, or try to think complexly. My brain was damaged, so why should I bother trying to do what I couldn't do?

Today, that still seems like the right decision. I had enough frustrations at the time; I didn't need more. Looking back, I see that I really did keep working on the problem, but in a backdoor way. No one got some blank paper and said "OK, now we'll practice writing fiction." Instead, I often played that child's game in which one person starts a story and the next one adds on.

4-27-86

I can't remember whose idea it was, a therapist or a friend, who suggested I try writing a journal longhand. Whoever it was, I am grateful. I'm a slow writer, and at first you could barely make out what I'd written. But I found writing a journal at the end of the day to be very relaxing. It also turned me into an editor; I write so slowly that I only put down the barest essentials so that now, editors ask me to add specifics, when before, they usually wanted me to chop. I had to accept that I wouldn't be able to write all of how I felt, but I could get down some. I never expected to get better or faster, but I did.

4-28-86

Something that must be quite puzzling to people close to brain-damaged adults is the lack of ability to make judgments. I heard of one man who was going through his closet, sorting out what to keep and what to give away. He just couldn't do it, and put some brand new things in the giveaway pile. I can sympathize. I might have done the same thing a few years ago. This inability to make judgments can make simple things like shopping impossible, especially in the U.S.A., where there are a lot of choices. Just yesterday, I had to put down a catalog. I just couldn't tell if 1) I liked the things; 2) if I needed it; and 3) did the price mean I couldn't get something else I needed?

I can see how a brain damaged adult might accrue wealth. She or he can't make up their mind on how to spend money. This is not my case, because being mobility impaired is expensive, but there's something to be said for that sort of indecision. It's thrifty.

4-28-86

Before I was disabled I reviewed books. To review books, one must be able to judge them. Fortunately, the first book I reviewed after I was disabled was a bore, and I knew when I was bored. Now to help me judge when I'm not bored, I read other people's faces more, ask other people's opinions, and try to gauge my reader's moods when she reads. Ultimately, it is my opinion of the book which I write down, but I do listen more, and I generally have most of my work read and critiqued by a class or my writers' group. I used to do these things, but now I'm more apt to do so.

4-26-86 (later)

Back when I'd only just gotten out of the hospital, and I'd been disabled just two years, there was an anthology being compiled of articles by disabled women for which I very much wanted to write. I tried to write for it, but even I, with my lousy judgment, could see that it was just no good. For one thing, the subject was too depressing. For another, I was brain damaged, and I wasn't making a whole lot of sense. This plunged me into despair unimaginable to the average person. I was an athlete who couldn't walk, a lover who couldn't make love (that at least usually comes back), and a writer who couldn't write. It didn't matter that I'd gotten a lot back: I'd lost my life, my future, and my writing ability, and nothing mattered.

Despite this awful despair that was present for five years, I kept getting up every morning trying to function, mostly because I had no choice. In a rehab, they won't let you lie around in bed. I tried that. My nurse felt that it was her fault, which it certainly wasn't. Then every single one of my rehab team came to convince me to me to get up. When I got out of the hospital, I didn't want my attendants to get into legal troubles, so I got out of bed.

Later, someone experienced in brain damage told me to slow down, that people who've been unable to work go overboard when they can again. I did go overboard, and I show no signs of slowing down, three years later. Not only did I think I was silent too long, but I'm much more aware of my own mortality now. I know I'm living on borrowed time, and I write a lot because I just don't know how long I'll be around.

5-2-86
I was talking with someone about comas and I told her that a large part of any gains I made had to do with my plain refusal to accept my prognosis. Not only did I refuse, but so did my family, and most of my friends. They knew

that someone who'd spent hours practicing one little maneuver in a ski turn so she could get certified would be able in muscle tone and willing mentally to spend time to become the best she can. They were right. Now that I've gotten back the ability to think complexly, I feel anything is possible. Because so much of my brain stem was destroyed (the part that transmits messages), it means that either those cells rejuvenated or some other brain tissue took over and is transmitting messages. It had to learn how to do it, and that's probably why my thoughts at first were simple and jumbled, and why parts of my body, when just starting to move, would move opposite to how I wanted. It didn't help that I was communicating in Morse code, and finger spelling, which have different syntaxes than American English.

5-17-86
When I first got out of the hospital, I fully expected that I'd get back my ability to walk. After all, I'd read enough of those "true-life drama" stories and figured it was only a matter of time. I wasn't that certain about getting my thinking and fiction back. (Authors Note. Or my ability to send my chi energy anywhere. I couldn't dream either. I rely on both abilities, but at the time, any talk about that would have sent me around the corner to a locked psych ward, so I couldn't say anything.) I'm glad there isn't the

commonplaceness around them. I'd have felt like such a failure, like I did for a while over not walking.

5-30-86

Over the past weekend, I experienced a flood of spirituality. When I had the stroke, I could not see any good whatever in it. I'd lost my ability to write for so long, and then to think complexly. I stopped believing in people having purposes in life; after all, every single one of mine had been taken away, how could I believe in anything but random events?

Once I got back the ability to think complexly and write lengthy fiction, I could start to believe in purpose again. Not as wholeheartedly as before, but I can see some good in the results of my insult. I am prolific since I am single and have nothing better to do. I write more now because there really wasn't any other thing I could do or study to eventually support myself. And all that time I would have spent doing athletics, I spend writing instead.

7-27-86

Was with a group of people today, and they were asking about problems with short-term memory. Mine, like many brain damaged people, was very bad at first. I asked people to write messages to others on a card taped to my chair.

My memory is much better now, but I still write things down. I keep a notebook in the house - things to do and things to put in my backpack.

Part of the reason I had problems with my memory in the hospital is that there's not much to remember in a day in a hospital or a nursing home.

10-02-86

I may be able to think complexly, but my brain still works quite differently now: I simply can't make the sort of snap decisions I used to. It takes me more time now. I'm also less flexible than I was. Say a doctor reschedules an appointment. I'm liable to show up for the original time. The most inexplicable and frustrating is a condition I saw called "flooding" in a movie about brain damage. There are times when I just can't talk, or times when something comes out of my mouth that is totally inappropriate. I think it must be associated with a particular part of the brain, because the flooding episodes vanished after I stopped breathing during a routine operation, and I've seen changes like that happen to others too.

DISABILITY 101: WHERE TO GO FOR HOUSING, WORK, AND BENEFITS

(Originally published in the 90's for *Sojourner: The Women's Forum.* It has been updated.)

Author's note: Social Security Disability-Income (SSDI) is technically not welfare. But, since so many newly disabled people don't have the vaguest idea about where to go for financial and other assistance, they think of welfare first. But the system is more complicated. This piece tries to provide some introductory information about getting benefits and support.

Fifteen years ago, when I had been disabled for only a few years, I realized that to keep my life simple the best thing would be to stay away from any agency that "helps" disabled people. This would have worked if I were a billionaire, but since I'm not, I really can't afford to do this. [Authors note. Things have totally changed. Most agencies really do help now, although I still advise getting everything in writing.] So, instead, I've tried to figure out which agency does what, and which ones are worth dealing with. Once you've been around awhile, you get to know the ins and outs. Nobody was born knowing all this stuff, so take it easy on yourself.

The first place I suggest people turn to is the Independent Living Centers (ILCs) or your state vocational rehabilitation commission (VR). You can usually find them in the phone book. Sometimes they get fancy and change the word order. Call 411. (You may get an exemption from phone charges for this call if you can't see or handle a phone book. Check with the phone company's business office or their disability services. No harm in asking, as my mom always said.)

When you reach the center or VR, ask to speak with someone in "Information and Referral." They will be able to tell you what services they offer. These may include:

• Lessons in Independent Living (IL)
• How to Find and Manage Personal Care Assistants (PCAs)
• Referral to Housing Agencies
• Support Groups
• Self-Advocacy

They don't use the name "Independent Living" for nothing. The workers at a good ILC or state VR will assume you're abler than any hospital ever will. They ask the impossible not only from you, but also from social service agencies, and often get it. The bad thing is that we are no longer in the '70s, and social services are simply not as accessible as they once were, I think because there are so many of us now.

WORK AND BENEFITS

The next thing to think about--well, you have to think about everything simultaneously, and that can be overwhelming. Let's take it gradually: work and/or getting benefits.

Catastrophic illness has a way of eating up savings, so money is probably important right now.

Because I was in a hospital for quite a long time, and because I had worked in the paid labor force long enough to receive disability "benefits," my Vocational Rehabilitation counselor from the Massachusetts Rehabilitation Commission found me and was able to help me out with benefits. VR benefits pay for school, computer expenses, work-related expenses, and some home modifications. Before you start jumping up and down with glee, though, remember that those overzealous bureaucrats are busy cutting VR budgets.

GETTING ON SSI OR SSDI

Everyone born in the USA is eligible for Supplemental Security Income (SSI) -- supposedly. SSI is based on the apparently old fashioned belief that we should assist those people who might need aid, including people who are old, sick, or pregnant. SSI isn't getting something for free. SSI is funded through state and federal taxes, which means that your parents, siblings, aunts, uncles, and other people you've never met have all paid tax to take care of a case exactly like yours. They paid into it for someone like you. It can take 18 to 24 months to receive your benefits, during which time you may be eligible for welfare.

Mostly anywhere in the United States, you can get a professional who specializes in getting SSDI for disabled people. They will charge you a percent of the back pay owed to you. You can also find a legal services lawyer or a disability law center in your area. Or, you can try to do it yourself (some people can handle it, although I tend to want to throw the phone against the wall) with the help of an Independent Living Skills specialist or a VR counselor.

SSDI is even "better" than SSI. The monetary benefits may be higher, although sometimes people who have never worked for pay get higher perks, and lawyers seem to feel that people on SSDI are better off because the money you're getting is based on your own work history. In other words, you're seen as having directly worked for it (like being a mom isn't work.) It used to take two or three months to receive benefits, but it now takes one to two years. Please realize that when you apply for SSDI, they will often say no the first time or two, in the hope that you will go away and stop bothering them. Also realize that some decision-makers still refuse to accept certain disabilities--like Chronic Fatigue Syndrome and Multiple Chemical Sensitivities. Occasionally, they give up and allow benefits for people with these disorders. Sometimes it's because a person's doctor can identify some other, allowable disability.

In recent years it's become clear that the government wants as many of us off of SSI and SSDI as possible. Just like we've heard the crazy stereotypes about welfare "queens" who drive Cadillacs, we've also heard the stories of perfectly able-bodied people who manage to draw disability checks for decades. However, the stories about companies bilking Medicaid for millions don't get equal coverage.

So many people, including government workers, believe that most SSDI recipients are "cheats." In any case, restrictions are getting ridiculous, and generate so much

busywork for the recipient that I'd like to say getting the
benefits is hardly worth the bother--except, of course, that
we need them to live and usually have no other place to
turn.

Here's one common scenario: trying to visit a doctor. First
of all, there's transportation. For the privilege of arriving
an hour late--but for free--at a doctor's appointment, you
have to call two days in advance, or better yet, two
months in advance, in order for someone to ask your
doctor's office to fax them a "PT-I." Your doctor will then
fill it out and send it to Medicaid. They reject it, for
unexplained reasons, and send it back to you. Then
another round of this begins. My current system is to take
the bus rather than rely on this "free" transportation that I
have no access to. I schedule all of my appointments in
the fall or spring. I tell the receptionist that if it rains hard
or snows, I may not be there. But since the new
wheelchairs (such as my trusty Quickie) don't stop dead in
their tracks when it rains anymore, this may change.

As for trying to get additional information about things like
SSI and SSDI, it can be an agonizingly slow process.
Funding from the offices that deal with these programs
has been sliced and diced, including programs getting
computers to disabled people. An advocate once
cheerfully told me that he thought some SSI bureaucratic

heads hated disabled people and didn't want to see them succeed.

Let me just note that state workers, the regular people in the SSI or SSDI offices, are not the bad guys here. Ever since a group of we disabled people camped out at the Massachusetts State House for nine days, I cannot regard them as such. They brought us flowers, platters of food, jokes, and encouragement. In short, I saw that they were mostly just working people doing the best they could under difficult circumstances. There are some who turn into babbling idiots when faced with a wheelchair, but that's not the majority. Talk to them reasonably (you'd be amazed at how few people do that), and don't assume the worker knows everything.

A LITTLE STREET ACTION

Of course, all these tactics may fail miserably, and a little street action, aimed at educating some agency, may be called for. Some activists declare that "being nice" leads nowhere, and simply do street actions. I myself am at heart one of those "nice" advocates, even though I've done my share of tying up traffic and offices. I generally know whom to complain to about what, and I don't waste my breath complaining to people who can't do anything.

Having activist activity behind you helps a lot because the people you negotiate with know that you can and will embarrass them. Coalitions I have worked with have scared up millions of dollars and helped pass legislation affecting healthcare and mass transportation nationally and even globally--thanks to the combined efforts of hundreds of "nice" advocates and less polite street actions.

BEFORE YOU GO: FROM BEDSORES TO BUMPY ROADS

Hey! You're almost outta here! There will probably be some spoilsports who will ask you if you're scared to leave the "protection" of the hospital. I think they were used to older patients for whom this is a big issue. Even so, it's a bit patronizing.

Come on! I was in my twenties! I couldn't WAIT!

One thing prevented people from leaving. They'd get too skinny, and start a bedsore. Bedsores are terrible, especially if they're on a paralyzed part. You may not feel them, but they won't heal as quickly as a non-paralyzed part. If they heal at all, that is. A man in my building had one that never really stayed healed.

There are all kinds of rumors about them, which I won't repeat. My advice, which this time I follow, is don't let them start in the first place.

If there is one thing you get out of this book, it is this: BE SERIOUS ABOUT BEDSORES!

Some days you will be lucky just to get out of bed. (Have pizza money hidden somewhere, and memorize the local pizza delivery phone number.) Ask whoever helps you to look you over for red marks on your skin. Slap some aloe or ready made cream on it immediately. Try to figure out where it came from. Usually it is splints and too tight shoes, and do your best to remedy this. Call your OT. Buy all your shoes bigger. Involve your Primary Care Doctor, your Case Manager, and whoever from your rehab is following your case. Years ago, it seemed there was no one to oversee things, but somewhere along the line this changed.

OK. There are a few things you should know that the professional rehabilitation experts probably don't know. For example, drunks and homeless people are going to be a lot friendlier. That is, if they weren't before. At first I thought I must look really bad. But then I found out that in certain cities, half the homeless population is disabled.

So 'they' see you as one of them. In the bad old days, you'd be ignored by nearly everyone except other disabled people and the homeless. At first I did not know how to deal with this. I guess that I was afraid of homeless people. That has changed, for many reasons, but one thing I learned when Governor Weld (a Republican who started off an enemy, but ended up an ally) tried to slash funding for PCAs: We are one pen-stroke away from homelessness.

But I'm getting sidetracked here. Let's talk about your apartment or shelter. Before you move in or back into your place, ask to have bumpers installed. Even if they just put stripping running down the edges of vulnerable walls, that will make you feel at home in your home. Also, put kick plates on vulnerable walls and doors, buy surge protectors, change doorknobs to handles, ask that the soap dish be moved closer and that the faucets be changed to a one handle type.

The units in my building were designed by an architect and a disabled person. I got very spoiled because my unit has raised electric plugs, low window handles, and a pulley system for the thermostat.

There are companies who specialize in this. They usually have the words ADA and Living or Home Modification in them. Check senior groups too.

One thing no one told me, with disastrous effects, is that electrical cords will get stuck on your footrests: you turn without knowing, and POP! There goes your phone on the floor, with a broken cord. Even worse, the cord to your hospital bed gets broken, so the bed is too high to get into, and the company can't come until next Tuesday. (Hint: electric beds generally have manual controls.)

A quad friend of mine told me he broke his foot by not noticing it had hit a wall. He then tried to turn, and well, let's say it's a good thing his wife is a nurse. I've sprained my paralyzed foot and stubbed toes or gotten mysterious cuts and bruises I can't explain.

If you are a walking amputee, this will probably happen to you. You'll be asleep, wake up terribly thirsty, and get up for a glass of water. Of course, you'll totally forget to put on your leg, and POW! Right on the floor.

If you wear a leg bag, chances are very good that one day you'll be in a hurry and your foot will slip into the bowl. Things like this happen. Keep a spray bottle filled with soap mixed with alcohol for these occasions, and know you'll have a laugh out of it someday.

SURVIVAL TACTICS

One way of dealing with budget cuts is to grow vegetables and medicinal herbs in your living room or community garden. The leaves of certain trees and houseplants are medicinal too. My theory--or should I say my great-grandmother the herbal medicinist's theory--is that an ounce of prevention is worth a pound of cure. The credit for my continuing hospital-free years (with a few exceptions) go everywhere, from the incredibly fresh foods of my youth, to my friends' care while in the hospital, my Haitian PCA whose care has been outstanding, western medications, complementary healthcare, and plenty of "simple" teas.

Another tip I wish I'd been told is: AIM FOR THE MIDDLE OF THE CURB CUT!! In the 80s, the few curb cuts that existed were badly made, and I spent a good amount of time in the road, on my face. Things have changed lately in Boston anyway, but there may be some old ones lurking around.

Only two things left. One is that your tires will screech when they get wet and you round a corner sharply. (Just don't tell Mayor Menino, OK? City Hall at night brings out the 11 year old tomboy in me, and I screech around the corners grinning wickedly.) And the other you need to know is this: Bumpy roads make you burp.

PART 3

YOU'RE OUT! GETTING AROUND AND OTHER POST-HOSPITAL CHALLENGES

(Previously published with some major changes) in *Hikane: The Capable Womon*, November 1991.)
Now your life can begin. Really. You can be sitting in one of the worst slums in the city, with zero money and most friends too terrified to visit you. I'm sure you'll have no trouble summing up all the horrible aspects of your life.

But you really are at the start of your new life. Life has pared you of a lot of things. It stinks, but there you are.

A few suggestions:
--Find other disabled people.

I once read a book called *The White Plague*. It described asylums for TB patients. One scene described older TB patients helping the newer ones. Even though the people lived 100 years ago, it was remarkably like present day interactions. The good thing about disability these days is that there are many groups focused narrowly. Start small, be comfortable. Stay narrowly focused for awhile. Hopefully, someday, we will hear your voice.

--Don't let your age or background limit you.
Elders are used to youngers teaching technology. It is really easy for me to be around twenty-something's. Not only are they the ages of my niece and nephews, but they have grown up around PWDs and have good manners. Not all of the advocates who "started" the Disability Rights Movement of the '70s have sterling silver backgrounds. Nor did all disabled people get that way because of alcohol abuse or illegal activity. How we all got here is way less important than what we do now.

--Know your rights.
This may be difficult because you may forget what they are, which is why you should carry booklets about the ADA with you.

--Get some credentials.

After a year of tangling with the Para transit in Boston, I was on it one day when the walkie-talkie crackled, ordering the driver to circle back and pick up the chairperson of the Transportation Committee. Light dawned.

So THAT was how to get a ride!

I'm happy to report that the current Para transit in Boston works fairly well now for everyone (at least compared to the worst days of our Para transit.)

I did take advantage of this patronage, but I needed to get around for my advocacy. I don't need it anymore, and the disability community has changed so much, I doubt I could do that again. But it's a tool I used, and one you might need for your own advocacy.

STATE HOUSE NURSING HOME: TAKING POLITICAL ACTION or MAKING TROUBLE IN MY ADOPTED HOMETOWN

Some of my best comedy was written in front of our governor's office, waiting to be arrested.

I guess that makes me an activist.

I'd always been careful to call myself an advocate. Being an advocate consists of making phone calls, pointing out code violations, finding out who to complain to about what, and doing it tactfully. (Because it seemed at the time that that was the only way to get anything done.)

But then the governor proposed taking away funding for our personal care assistants. This is roughly equivalent to the police coming into your house in the wee hours of the morning and dragging you to jail.

I tend to think of myself as relatively harmless, and I was totally outraged. If I didn't have assistants, I couldn't live in my own apartment. That left living with my parents in New Hampshire (impossible, their house was barely accessible), the streets of Boston (ha), a nursing home (where they sometimes force drugs on you, and staph infections run rampant -- between the two, I'd probably die), or jail. Jail seemed the best alternative. So there I was, at the State House, beeping my horn and yelling. Looking over my shoulder constantly. I needn't have bothered being so careful. As time passed, I realized how safe I was.

Walkers, wheelchairs, canes and crutches are lethal, and I came to trust that I would be defended if need be, and not just by other disabled people either. There were a lot of state workers who, disgruntled by the governor's policy of making them work two weeks without pay, told us they hoped we got our way.

The first demo, at which people were sure they'd get arrested, was held on a fairly warm May day in front of the governor's office. I stayed toward the back of the demo so that I could slip away if need be. But the demo got bigger and bigger and I could see the commitment of the people there: mild-mannered types that you'd never ever see at anything radical; the usual activists displaying far more fervor than I'd ever seen; and some people who, despite having more fragile bodies than I do, and mine has many frailties, were there, being vocal or at least letting their displeasure be known. I realized something remarkable was happening, and all that commitment infected me too.

So I signed one of the "in an emergency, contact..." forms and made my way to the front with the other arrestees. Well, we sat around and waited. We had a speak out, using assistants to give voice or to read spelled out messages, told stories and jokes, and listened to a woman play her recorder. But mostly, we waited.

This is how I came to write comedy in front of the governor's office. It was to be my second gig, and until then, I didn't think of performing as anything more than a passing thing. The longer I sat, the funnier the jokes seemed to get. I realized that here was a weapon "they" couldn't take away, not even if I was paralyzed and speechless again. "They" could cut the Para transit all they wanted; I could take the bus or drive my wheelchair to our local women's bookstore where I perform. And if anyone took offense, I could say it was just a joke.

Our first demo fizzled out. So we went home and tried to think up things to do next. I was in on several planning meetings, vowed secrecy, and even now am not sure what I can and can't say, but there were a lot of people risking jobs, funding for their agency, and the tiny gains we had made.

But there didn't seem to be any choice. We decided to set up a symbolic nursing home at the State House. Setting it up was easy. There were no security checks, and since few people ever noticed people with disabilities back then, getting cots in required no subterfuge. We did it in shifts, so out of nine days and nights, I did six days. A lot of people from my building were there doing shifts because it was close and we live on an accessible bus route. Some of it was fun, like getting to know each other better, or trading jokes with the lone officer they had guarding us, or when one of the state worker's offices sent us a plate of food.

Most of it was boring, but even so, a little too nerve-wracking for me. Rather patronizingly, they don't usually arrest wheelchair users yet in Boston, but you never know when anyone will change her/his mind.

It took the press and the governor six days to finally acknowledge our presence, but once that happened, the media was upon us.

Update: We did our action in 1991. Sometimes it seems like "they" are out to get us; however, our governor created the post of liaison to the disabled community in '92. I went to the ceremony. During it I realized part of me was no longer outside the law. It felt strange.

Best of all is the difference in how "they" see us. Shortly after this the mainstream press referred to someone as having the "persistence of people with disabilities at the State House." Too, on the following July 4th three million tourists and I were downtown to see the fireworks. Just as I started heading for a curb cut, a man pulled into the space. Seeing me, he pulled out again and parked elsewhere. He got out, put his hands in the air and said sadly, "I'm sorry, I really didn't see you." Quite a difference from five years ago, when most drivers just ignored us.

Many years ago, before I became disabled, I had to walk to work to a ski area in the winter. My breath turned to ice as I watched cars zip up the hill I had to climb. Just then I glanced up to see a flock of wild geese fly by. After becoming disabled, I never thought I'd feel that free again without being able to walk. But I do get that feeling now when I'm out picketing, talking about silly laws, even just telling another disabled person that s/he has more power than s/he thinks.

WHEELCHAIR FLYING: MY FAVORITE SPORT

After seeing me perform stand-up comedy from my wheelchair, people ask if I get nervous. I laugh at that one. Nervous is standing at the top of a slalom course at an international race, thirteen years old and the only girl on the team, knowing that how you ski will decide the team's fate. When I turned fourteen, I went down a race course composed mostly of rutted ice, skied over to my parents, and told them I'd never race again.

I had always dreamt of being a national team member. A friend of mine had been on a 1950s Swiss team, and she'd shown me her medal and pictures. I had wanted that.

But what started out fun turned into a nightmare. I kept losing by tenths of a second. My competitive nature and good skiing form just weren't quite enough. Finally, I decided to become a ski instructor like my mother and father. Teaching turned out to be a wonderful choice for me. I had the aggressiveness and strength to survive in an all-male professional environment, I loved entertaining people, and teaching let me be around children, whom I really enjoyed. In time I graduated from college and started working with computers. I drifted away from teaching after ten seasons.

Two years later, I had a stroke.

Now I indulge in a sport few people have tried--flooring my motorized wheelchair. I call it wheelchair flying. Wheelchair flying takes place on an asphalt path around a bicyclists pond. (Authors note: Which Jamaica Pond no longer is.) I startle people as I zoom by them at a full-out 7 mph. Part of the high of this sport is that people get a new slant on wheelchairs and wheelchair users. One time, a little kid pointed at my chair and said,

"Look, Mom, can you get me one?"

Wheelchair flying gives me the freedom to... well, stretch my "legs." While negotiating the able-bodied world, I must constantly stretch or squeeze myself. I strain to hear and see, speak slowly so I'm understood, and force myself to be polite to people with patronizing attitudes (they don't know better, although I try to educate them). I'm carried in and out of some places, and in others maneuver the chair very, very carefully to avoid hitting cars, furniture, or the many people who think they have the right to walk directly in my path.

When I'm wheelchair flying, I don't need to deal with any of that. The pond is known for fast runners and bicyclists. Parents hold their children's hands. Runners keep their dogs on leashes. And I leave room on both sides of me so bikes can get by. Wheelchair flying there is like driving a motorcycle down a winding back road in a country where they drive on the "wrong" side. Now that's a challenge.

I wouldn't do this if I had no reflexes, or couldn't see or hear well with correction. And I make certain my seat belt is fastened. Although I just laugh when I'm told adaptive athletics are dangerous. Give me a break. I'm already in a wheelchair. And flying fine.

THE QUESTIONS: Q&A WITH THE AUTHOR

Since everyone asks the same questions, and I get tired of answering them, I'm going to interview myself. If you think of any new ones, I may think about it, but not too long or hard. The stroke happened 28 years ago, after all.

If you insist in asking questions about that time of my life when I was more, you think, "like you," I may start asking you what was the most painful period of your life and ask you deeply personal questions that force you to relive your divorce or the death of someone quite close.

Back when I was still on medication and hating myself, those questions made me feel awful. I have no idea how they would make me feel now, but I'm not eager to find out. All my life, I've never understood what difference it makes anyway. I have so many disabled friends that I have forgotten who has what. It doesn't make any difference in who they are now.

If you are so interested you MUST know, examine your reasons. Is it that you need to know I was born "that way" so you can breathe a sigh of relief that you missed that one? Do you need to know the "cause" so you can delude yourself into believing that if you do such and so, you won't become disabled?

Do you only respond to the person I was, and if so, why?

Q, When did you...?
A. June 27, 1981.
(Which also happens to be the anniversary of the 1969 Stonewall riots. And on June 27, 2005, Eric Rofes, a gay activist author, died. I died in 1981, but I was revived.)

Q. What happened?
A. I had a type of stroke.

Q. A stroke! WEREN'T YOU KIND OF YOUNG FOR ONE?
A. No. Babies have strokes.
Actually the kind I had, an AVM, or Arterial Venus Malformation, usually happens in young adulthood. I was born with a malformed blood vessel.

Q. When did you have yours?
A. When I was 27.

Q. Did you have any idea?
A. For most of my life, no. The year I had the AVM, I knew something was quite wrong, but years of eating game and garden fresh vegetables and being an athlete

took over. I was having tests done, including blood pressure, EEG, and EKG, but they all came out just fine.

When you think of it, it's amazing I didn't injure myself long before this. I started downhill racing at eight. I white-water kayaked. I loved to go backpacking in the White Mountains by myself. I have done more stupid things in my life (trading seats on a moving chairlift going over a ravine, skiing 60 mph inches behind someone going equally as fast, need I go on?) Now it seems to me that I got the only destiny in store. Every doctor in those first years who examined me asked me how I ever walked on those knees.

Q. So it affected your left side?
A. It affected everything. I was totally paralyzed and speechless, plus it affected my ability to think.

Q. Weren't you scared?
A. To be scared implies understanding of the situation. I did not. Once I did, I thought all I had to do was be patient. After all, my mother had faced not being expected to walk twice or speak again when she had childhood polio. Her close friends never knew. As a medic, my father had saved several people who surpassed their predicted fates. I just assumed I would recover completely. What I

was very afraid about was losing my ability to write and my 'rainbow,' which was my term for 'chi.'

Q. And you didn't give up.
A. Try that sometime.

Q. Still, I don't know if I could have handled it as well.
A. Sure you would. You'd be surprised at how much the body can take. And you'd almost certainly be a better patient!

Q. Will you ever get better?
A. I am better.

THE END

BIBLIOGRAPHY

Grollman, Earl. Caring and Coping When Your Loved One is Seriously Ill. Boston: Beacon Press, 1995. Print. (Note: I love this man's writing!)

Grollman, Earl. In Sickness and in Health: How to Cope When Your Loved One is Ill. Boston: Beacon Press, 1987. Print.

Hathaway, Katherine Butler. The Little Locksmith: A Memoir. New York: The Feminist Press at CUNY, 2000. Print.

"Listen to Our Stories: Words, Pictures, and Songs by Young People with Disabilities." Ed. Hillyer, Linda. 2006, 2008 <http://www.listentoourstories.com>.

Jacobs, Ruth H. Be an Outrageous Older Woman. New York: Harper Paperbacks, 1997. Print.

Nielsen, Kim. The Radical Lives of Helen Keller. New York: NYU Press, 2004. Print.

Panzarino, Connie. The Me in the Mirror. Berkeley, CA: Seal Press, 1994. Print.

Rodman, John S., R. Ernest Sosa, Cynthia Seidman, and Rory Jones, Eds. No More Kidney Stones: The Experts Tell You All You Need to Know about Prevention and Treatment. NJ: Wiley, 2007. Print.

Zion, Leonard. Finding Another Voice: Moments of Wonder. Moments of Wonder Press, 2007. Available for print purchase from http://www.lulu.com/product/paperback/finding-another-voice-~-moments-of-wonder/724768

RESOURCES

BOSTON AREA

Amethyst Center for Healing
259 Elm Street
Somerville, MA
617-591-9200
Acupuncture, chiropractic, movement therapy, naturopathic and more.
Massachusetts only, ask your doctor for a referral.

Boston Women's Fund
http://www.bostonwomensfund.org
Donate to fund start-ups for women and girls.

http://www.Linkpink.com
Find lgbt-friendly businesses in the NE area.

http://www.mass-match.org
Several agencies banded together to get adaptive equipment to people who need it.

http://www.Newbalance.com

They can be pricey, but they have an outlet store, and regular sales. They usually have good treads but let the buyer beware. I got one Velcro fastened sneak with no tread whatsoever.

http://www.mbta.com
The MBTA Ride
1-877-765-7433
Talk about love-hate relationships! Most of the time, they are just fine, but it will take years for me to forgive them for wasting 2 hours I could have spent with my 86 year old mother who died the next month. She would have told me to forget it, and I will someday, but not yet.

Tobias & Batitte (hearing aids)
617-426-2226
(MA only. Ask your doctor for a referral if you live elsewhere.)

NATIONAL

http://www.easterseals.com
The Easter Seals in Massachusetts is a dream, providing technical training, job support, dignified fundraising, and

summer camps. Apparently, each state is different, but check it out. Their ideal is impressive.

http://www.enemeez.com
The mere mention of its' name usually gets nervous laughter, but it changed MY life.

http://www.freecycle.org
The name pretty much says it all. People offer stuff free, hopefully unclogging a landfill or two. Be prepared to haul it away.

http://www.ncil.org
Go here to find Independent Living Centers in your area. They are a good resource for all People with Disabilities, but especially for those floundering with everything at once.

http://www.dlc-ma.org/_manual/LASE_manual.htm
"Planning for Life After Special Education: A Transition Services Online Manual" edited by the Disability Law Center, in conjunction with the Federation for Children with Special Needs, the Institute for Community Inclusion, and Massachusetts Advocates for Children
http://rsa.ed.gov/view_info.cfm
Use this link to find the various rehabilitation agencies in your state.

http://smartasscripple.blogspot.com/
Not everyone will appreciate his humor, but I go there
frequently any time I need a good laugh. Thanks Mike.

http://www.silverscript.com
My Medicare Part D prescription plan, which has not
produced an ounce of busywork, a minor miracle.

ACKNOWLEDGEMENTS

This is the best part for an author: publicly thanking everyone who has helped you write, including the electrician who bounded down Heath Street to retrieve the mock baseball I used to use as a hand grip to steer my wheelchair.

This is also the part that fills me with dread, because I know I'll forget someone very important who gave me something essential to the writing of this book. If that's you, I'm very sorry. I could blame my brain damage, but I like my father's reasoning better. He said older people are so good at thinking that the thoughts go by too fast to catch on to. So here goes, and please forgive me that I forgot people.

First, to my first publisher, Mona Barbera of Dos Monos Press, who emailed me through the rough spots; Maida Tilchen for editing and manuscript preparation, Tom Hubschman and Ellen Larson of Savvy Press who helped me change course midstream so I could get published faster; Russ, Dave and Jeannette Dearborn, my cheerleaders; Lisa Dearborn, who listened to my vague longings and designed a great cover; Pat Couglin and family; Nancy Taylor and family; Stephanie Poggi; Damian

Marcotte ; Loie Hayes and family; Deb Cavicchi; Tiyo Sallah-El; Angela; Chris Guilfoy; Gert Dearborn; Ron Aruda; Joan Gay; Gwen and Ed Raswyck; Myrna Greenfield; Shelley; Sherrard Hamilton; Warren Garner; Meizhu Lui; Joanne O'Connell; Amy Hasbrouck; Clair Robeson; Helene Newburg; Mary Kennedy; and Barbara Beckwith.

Mike Riegle's death in 1992 spurred this book, but the world wasn't ready for it yet. He thought I was lucky because I had an obvious job of educating people about disability. I wasn't too happy about it then, but he was right! Now, finally, there are so many of us now to do things that I can focus on writing and stand-up, so to speak.

Mass Rehab Commission (especially Susan Marcus-Alter); Tenth Mountain vets; Boston Center for Independent Living (especially Bill Henning and Karen Schneiderman); Boston Public Library (especially L. Harris); Back of the Hill Apartments staff (both past and present); Easter Seals of Massachusetts (where I polished this book, and Katrina Parker and Peter Litchfield patiently taught me techie tips); Perkins Talking Book Library (especially Rachel Gould); Mary K. Callahan; wheelchairrecycler.com; and the Amethyst Center in Somerville. Even the MBTA and the Ride! I've made a lot of jokes at your expense, but you've come a long, long way, even if you kicked and screamed at first.

Working at the papers *Gay Community News* and *Sojourner: The Women's Forum*; the bookstores Crones' Harvest and New Words; and the philanthropic Boston Women's Fund have given me the opportunity to meet semi-famous and well-known people. So thanks to them for taking me seriously and I hope our paths cross again.

ABOUT THE AUTHOR

Carrie Dearborn is a writer, comedian, and advocate on disability issues. Her articles, essays and book reviews have appeared in *Sojourner: The Women's Forum; Equal Times; The New England Women's Yellow Pages; Gay Community News; Lambda Book Report; Jamaica Plain Gazette; This Brain Has a Mouth; Disability Rag;* as well as the Farrar, Straus and Giroux anthology, *Whatever It Takes: Women on Women's Sport.*

A former computer operator specialist and downhill ski instructor, Dearborn was 27 in 1981 when she had a stroke resulting from an Arterial Venus Malformation. One of the first AVM stroke survivors, she was kept alive by machines for one month, and spent seven months voiceless. She lived in the Boston Center for Independent Living Transitional Housing, and now lives in the community and uses a power wheelchair. Dearborn has had gigs doing "sit-down comedy" at neighborhood, heath care, disability, and gay and lesbian groups.

Dearborn is an advocate for people with disabilities on issues ranging from transportation access to health care issues. She has served on the board of the Boston Center for Independent Living, and was an advisor for many

MBTA projects. In 1991, as part of the Disability Rights Movement, she joined 50 other wheelchair users at a 9-day 'lie-in" at the Massachusetts State House, after the governor tried to slashed funding for personal care attendants. The funding was restored.

She has a degree from New England College in Henniker, NH. She lives in Jamaica Plain, Massachusetts with her caregiver of 26 years. She is a member of the National Writers Union.

CONNECT WITH CARRIE DEARBORN ONLINE
Please write to me at disabilityprimer@aol.com

② HP
8/14

Made in the USA
Charleston, SC
05 February 2014